SECRETS OF SLEEP

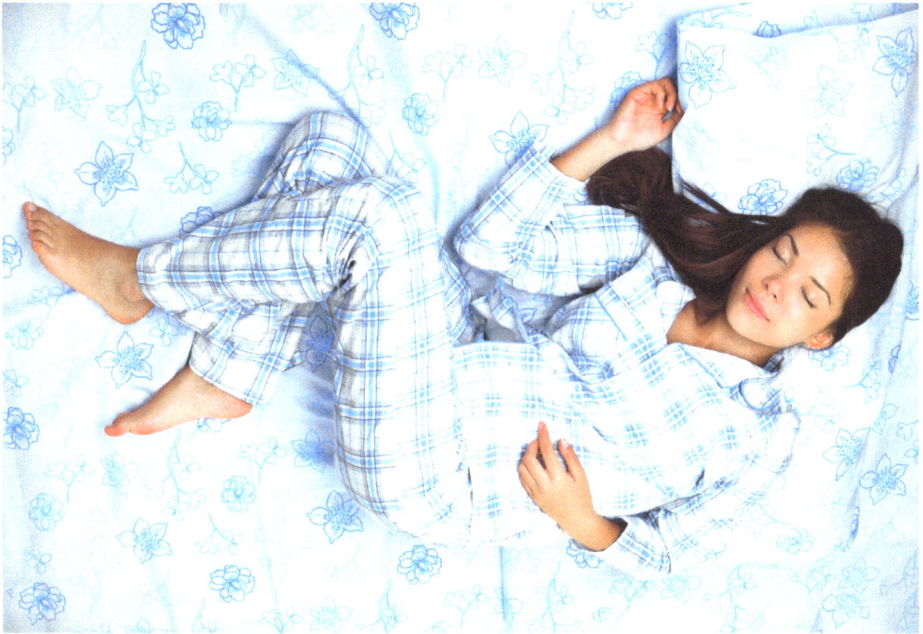

"All you need to know about a good night's rest."

Elle Smith

DISCLAIMER

The information contained in "SECRETS OF SLEEP" and its components, is meant to serve as a comprehensive collection of strategies that the author of this Ebook has done research about. Summaries, strategies, tips and tricks are only recommendations by the author, and reading this Ebook will not guarantee that one's results will exactly mirror the author's results.

The author of this Ebook has made all reasonable efforts to provide current and accurate information for the readers of this Ebook. The author and its associates will not be held liable for any unintentional errors or omissions that may be found.

The material in the Ebook may include information by third parties. Third party materials comprise of opinions expressed by their owners. As such, the author of this Ebook does not assume responsibility or liability for any third party material or opinions.

The publication of third party material does not constitute the author's guarantee of any information, products, services, or opinions contained within third party material. Use of third party material does not guarantee that your results will mirror our results. Publication of such third party material is simply a recommendation and expression of the author's own opinion of that material.

Whether because of the progression of the Internet, or the unforeseen changes in company policy and editorial submission guidelines, what is stated as fact at the time of this writing may become outdated or inapplicable later.

TABLE OF CONTENTS

Introduction   5

The Mystery Of Sleep   7

Why I Can't Sleep   9

How Much Sleep Do You Need?   13

Top Secrets To A Good Night's Sleep   15

Massage - a vital key to having a good night's rest   23

Passion flower   29

Importance Of A Good Night's Sleep   31

Foods You Should Not Eat When Going To Bed   37

Take Home Message   39

Your Worry List   40

INTRODUCTION

One in five Americans sleeps less than six hours a night—a trend that can have serious personal health consequences. Sleep deprivation increases the risk for some chronic health problems, including obesity, diabetes, and heart disease. If you have trouble sleeping, we have just compiled some strategies that can help you get more sleep in this Ebook. Read on!

Secrets of Sleep

CHAPTER 1

THE MYSTERY OF SLEEP

It's where our brains travel to every night, it's out of our voluntary control, and we often complain that we don't get enough of it. Sleep is the mysterious shift in consciousness that our bodies require every day. It's vital for our health and well-being, but its importance goes far beyond that, sleep is something that we can't live without. Not only do we function worse when we don't get enough quality sleep, but it can lead to long-term health problems. That's why if we're having sleep problems, it's important we do all that we can to rectify these difficulties and restore quality sleep into our lifestyles.

Secrets of Sleep

CHAPTER 2

WHY I CAN'T SLEEP

If you have ever kept asking over and over again, "why can't I sleep?" you know just how aggravating it can be. Not only is it annoying when you can't sleep, but you are not going to have a very good day because you are going to be tired and crabby, and will not able to function properly. If you can't sleep at night, it may be for a number of reasons.

Stress is one of the biggest reasons why many people don't sleep well, and the best thing to do about this is to find out what the cause is, then look for ways to eliminate it. If stress is not the problem, you may not be sleeping for other reasons. Some of the things that can cause sleepless nights include:

Being Over-Stimulated: If you are too active before bedtime, it is going to take a while for your body and your mind to be able to wind down. Try not to do any physical activities just before going to bed, and do not get involved in anything that is going to stimulate your brain, even if it's a really good book. You want your body and mind to be relaxed when you are ready to go to sleep at night.

Eating and Drinking: You should never have a heavy meal before going to bed. Your body is going to have to digest the food you eat before it can even think about starting to settle down for the night. You should also avoid certain beverages, especially any that contain caffeine and alcoholic beverages. If you do need a snack at bed time, make it something very light, and just have a glass of water to wash it down.

Smoking: If you are a smoker, it is a good idea to quit, for many reasons. Not only is smoking terrible for your overall health, but it is also something that can keep you awake at night. Nicotine is a stimulant, and those who think they can't get to sleep without a cigarette are actually making a huge mistake because it is going to keep them awake rather than help them get to sleep.

Stress and worry: This is another reason why people can't go to sleep. It could very well be the most common given the way things are everywhere. Work related stress, family issues, these are the issues that cause you to worry which leads to stress and then, not being able to sleep.

Equally it may be due to a poor mattress which should in fact allow air to circulate, be supportive and it should be noted that springs avoided in favour of a gel or foam mattress. These of course need to be kept clean, aired and changed after some years, given the sweat, skin and bed bugs. These are just a few of the most common reasons why some people can't get to sleep. If you keep asking yourself, "why can't I sleep?" and you have ruled out all of the above reasons, it may be time to talk to your doctor and find out what is making you unable to sleep at night. The sooner you find out what is causing the problem, the sooner you can deal with it and start sleeping better.

Sleep and your health

As mentioned, lack of sleep can contribute towards many health problems, and this has been shown in studies involving night-shift workers.

The risks for heart disease and type 2 diabetes are increased, and there is a growing body of evidence showing that poor sleep patterns are directly linked to being overweight and obesity. There are many reasons for this, including low serotonin and consequently melatonin levels which make you more likely to eat more sugary foods and refined carbohydrates because these foods increase levels of serotonin.

Lack of sleep has also been shown to increase levels of the hunger hormone ghrelin, which stimulates appetite and makes us feel hungry, and it decreases levels of the satiety hormone leptin, which gives us that satisfied feeling after eating that prompts us to stop eating.

CHAPTER 3

HOW MUCH SLEEP DO YOU NEED?

On average, most adults seem to need around 7-8 hours' sleep per night; though this can vary from person to person. As we grow older, our sleep patterns change, and as we go through life stages, we tend to get less and less sleep. Older adults tend to sleep less, not because they need less sleep, but because we're more likely to experience disturbed sleep as we grow older.

On average

» New-born babies sleep up to 18-21 hours per day
» 3-5-year-olds sleep 11-13 hours per day
» Pre-teens need 11 hours
» Teenagers need 9-11 hours

On average women are more likely to experience insomnia and sleep disturbances than men.

Secrets of Sleep

CHAPTER 4

TOP SECRETS TO A GOOD NIGHT'S SLEEP

Tired of feeling tired? Here are some simple tips to help you get to sleep.

After a night spent tossing and turning, you wake up feeling like a couple of the Seven Dwarves: Sleepy and Grumpy. As we all know, restless nights and weary mornings can become more frequent as we get older and our sleep patterns change—which often begins around the time of menopause when hot flashes and other symptoms awaken us.

We all have trouble sleeping from time to time, but when insomnia persists day after day, it can become a real problem. Beyond making us tired and moody, a lack of sleep can have serious effects on our health, increasing our propensity for obesity, heart disease, and type 2 diabetes.

If you've been having trouble falling asleep or staying asleep, you may have turned to sleep medications in search of more restful slumber. However, these drugs can have side effects—including appetite changes, dizziness, drowsiness, abdominal discomfort, dry mouth, headaches, and strange dreams. A recent study in the British Medical Journal associated several hypnotic sleep aids, including zolpidem (Ambien) and temazepam (Restoril), with a possible increased risk of death (although it did not confirm how much of the risk was related to these drugs).

You don't need to avoid sleep aids if you absolutely need them, but before you turn to pills, try these twelve tips to help you get a better night's sleep:

1. Exercise

Going for a brisk daily walk won't just trim you down, it will also keep you up less often at night. Exercise boosts the effect of natural sleep hormones such as melatonin. A recent study found that postmenopausal women who exercised for about three-and-a- half hours a week had an easier time falling asleep than women who exercised less often. Just watch the timing of your workouts.

Exercising too close to bedtime can be stimulating – a morning workout is ideal. Exposing yourself to bright daylight first thing in the morning will help the natural circadian rhythm.

2. Reserve bed for sleep and sex

Don't use your bed as an office for answering phone calls and responding to emails. Also, avoid watching late-night TV there. Your bed needs to be a stimulus for sleeping, not for wakefulness.

3. Keep it comfortable

Television isn't the only possible distraction in your bedroom. Ambience can affect your sleep quality too. Make sure your bedroom is as comfortable as possible. Ideally, you want a quiet, dark, cool environment. All of these things promote sleep onset.

4. Consider The Lavender Essential Oil

Lavender is one of the well-known natural remedy for insomnia. In fact, it has been used for a range of medicinal uses over the years and has continued to be a favourite of the cosmetic industry owing to its fragrance and its beneficial effects upon the skin.

In relation to sleeping, it has been shown to depress the central nervous system causing the person using it to become more relaxed. This relaxation helps in the process of sleep.

Before bed, spray your pillow and face with lavender diluted in distilled water, take a few deep breaths, inhaling lavender directly from the vial or a drop on a tissue, or place dried lavender buds in a sachet in your pillow case.

5. Start a sleep ritual

When you were a child and your mother read you a story and tucked you into bed every night, this comforting ritual helped lull you to sleep. Even in adulthood, a set of bedtime rituals can have a similar effect.

Rituals help signal the body and mind recognize it's coming up to time for sleep. Take a bath, or listen to calming music to unwind before bed.

6. Eat—but not too much

A grumbling stomach can be distracting enough to keep you awake, but so can an overly full belly. Avoid eating a big meal within two to three hours of bedtime. If you're hungry right before bed, eat a small healthy snack (such as an apple with a slice of cheese or a few healthy crackers) to satisfy you until breakfast.

7. Avoid alcohol and caffeine

If you do have a snack before bed, wine and chocolate shouldn't be part of it. Chocolate contains caffeine, which is a stimulant. Surprisingly, alcohol has a similar effect. "People think it makes them a little sleepy, but it's actually a stimulant, and it disrupts sleep during the night," Dr. Carlson says. You should stay away from anything acidic (such as citrus fruits and juices) or spicy, which can give you heartburn.

8. Consume more honey and milk

Honey and milk have both been traditionally used as remedies for insomnia and sleeplessness. Individually, they are both effective, but the effects are strengthened when taken together. Honey is one of the rare sugary foods causing a controlled increase in the amount of insulin being secreted, which also promotes tryptophan to be released into the brain.

Tryptophan is normally converted into serotonin, which induces a feeling of relaxation. Furthermore, serotonin is commonly converted to melatonin, a well-researched sleep aid. Through that rather confusing chemical pathway, honey and milk can be used to reduce sleeplessness.

9. De-stress

The bills are piling up, and your to-do list is a mile long. Daytime worries can bubble to the surface at night. Stress is a stimulus. It activates the fight-or-flight hormones that work against sleep. Give yourself time to wind down before bed. Learning some form of the relaxation response can promote good sleep and may also reduce daytime anxiety. Another method of relaxation is deep breathing exercises. Inhale slowly and deeply, and then exhale.

An urge to move your legs, snoring and a burning pain in your stomach, chest, or throat are symptoms of three common sleep disrupters—restless leg syndrome, sleep apnoea, and gastroesophageal reflux disease or GERD (Gastroesophageal Reflux Disease). If these symptoms are keeping you up at night or making you sleepy during the day, see your doctor for an evaluation.

11. Meditation

Mindfulness meditation helps fight insomnia, improves sleep. Now, a small study suggests that mindfulness meditation — a mind-calming practice that focuses on breathing and awareness of the present moment — can truly help.

Mindfulness meditation involves focusing on your breathing and then bringing your mind's attention to the present without drifting into concerns about the past or future. It helps you break the train of your everyday thoughts to evoke the relaxation response, using whatever technique feels right to you.

12. Well-maintained mattress

There is nothing more comforting than coming home after a long hard day and having a good night's sleep on your foam mattress. It is important to have the perfect mattress to sleep on allowing you to wake up feeling refreshed and full of energy which in turn helps you cope with your daily stresses. You should shop around when buying a mattress to find a mattress that suits your specific needs, and that also gives your body the support it needs when resting. Ensure you spray your mattress, pillows, and beddings for bugs and dust mites regularly – as they are hindrance factor to a good night rest.

CHAPTER 5

MASSAGE - A VITAL KEY TO HAVING A GOOD NIGHT REST

Massage is one of the vital things that helps in relaxing one's self, and the one I recommend to you is the Lomi Lomi Massage.

Lomi Lomi massage is based on the belief that a human being's cell memories will either improve or negatively affect the whole condition of the body.

When the body lacks harmony, the result is pain emotionally, spiritually, mentally and physically. Sickness is as a result of tension, which effectively leads to physical resistance blocking the movement of energy. The Hawaiian Lomi Lomi massage therapy helps in releasing this tension.

HOW TO PERFORM A LOMI LOMI MASSAGE

Choose your oils.

You can choose to use water-based oil as it is easier to clean afterward. Remember you are doing it at home, so maybe your husband will or wife can help you out with this procedure. The key performers with this massage are the ingredients. Jojoba oil, grapeseed, or almond are all recommended for this massage, with a couple of drops of the lavender essential oil. Sesame oil is good during cold seasons as it gently warms up the body. In summer months, you may want to use coconut oil as it naturally helps to cool the body.

Before you start the procedure, confirm that the person having the massage does not have allergies to products like lavender or almond oil. There are always alternatives to nut-based oils, for example, evening primrose, jasmine or safflower oils. Avocado oil is another alternative, but this is a heavier oil and is perhaps better suited to more mature skin.

Create the right atmosphere

This is very important as location is everything to relaxation. A cold room or a room where external noise can interrupt you zoning out to a space for relaxation should of course be avoided.

You can prepare the room for the massage space by having some essential oils sprinkled around, burning incense or pampering with fresh flowers in an atmosphere of low, ambient lighting. If the massage recipient loves music, you could have some soothing background music.

Channeling the positive energy

The massage recipient should be laying face down, ask them to take a couple of deep breaths. Proceed by placing your hands on their back where it corresponds to the heart. Your goal is to channel positive energy down from your heart and coming through both of your hands.

Muscle warm up

It is important to warm up the muscles as you begin a massage just like a seasoned athlete would. You can start with long, light flowing strokes on the surface, working more deeply into the muscles as you progress. Remember relaxation is key, and a gentle build-up will allow the person to feel comfy and give them time to zone out of every day life.

Move smoothly

It's vital that a calm, almost meditative mental state is achieved in order to bring the desired calmness to the recipient. Use soothing, flowing movements using both your hands in fluid, long sweeps. Remember to use enough oil so as to avoid causing unpleasant friction, but not too much.

Methodically work through the body

Start at the back and gradually work through the rear of the arms, the neck, the legs, ending at the feet. If the person receiving the massage is comfortable with a front massage, address the legs upwards to the arms, and chest.

Stimulating reflex points located in the feet and hands releases endorphins which bring a whole body feel-good effect. Always try to achieve order in terms of what areas you address, as connecting areas of the body is more natural, rather than changing from one location to another. Equally, the sense of oozing the daily stresses out of the body is achieved by this flow of movement.

Use your intuition

Listen carefully to the body and if an area goes red or tenses up, give that section some extra work. There are definitely some areas that are no-go zones like the stomach as it can feel too intimate.

Always seek the opinion of the person receiving the massage before you start and always avoid the surprise element by keeping your movements fluid. Likewise if an area offers more relaxation to the recipient, go with the flow giving deeper therapy to offer maximum benefit of your 'loving hands' therapy.

Finish in a nurturing way

Cool down the person's muscles with relaxing, long strokes and finish with one more energy balance just like you started – just as the traditional Huna Lomi Lomi massage was designed to do.

CHAPTER 6

PASSION FLOWER

As its name suggests, passion flower is a plant. Passion flower is a climbing shrub native to the tropical parts of the United States which produces a beautiful, delicate flower that develops into a large, fleshy fruit. It is used as a remedy for different ailments, including sleep deprivation. The chemicals in passion flower have calming, sleep inducing, anxiety and muscle spasm relieving effects.

Drinking a passion flower tea an hour before bedtime might help improve sleep quality.

If you're an insomniac, passion flower is even more effective when combined with other herbs. The combination of passion flower, valerian, hops, and lemon balm is a common formula used for inducing sleep. To use passion flower for sleep, look for it combined with hops and valerian, and possibly with lemon balm as well. Since these preparations are sold in various strengths, take the dose recommended on the bottle as a starting dose. Stress, anxiety, and poor sleep don't have to rule your life. You can get these problems under control with natural medicine.

In many cases, a more comprehensive approach, using other nutrients, dietary changes, and lifestyle changes will enhance the effectiveness of herbal anxiety remedies like passion flower.

CHAPTER 7

IMPORTANCE OF A GOOD NIGHT'S SLEEP

Consistently getting a good night's sleep is one of the best things you can do for your health. However, many of us are often so busy with work, family, social obligations and errands that we end up sacrificing sleep to fit everything in.

Here are 10 reasons why good sleep is important.

1. Poor Sleep Can Make You Fat

Poor sleep is strongly linked to weight gain. People with short sleep duration tend to weigh significantly more than those who get adequate sleep.In fact, short sleep duration is one of the strongest risk factors for obesity.

In one massive review study, children and adults with short sleep duration were 89% and 55% more likely to become obese, respectively. The effect of sleep on weight gain is believed to be mediated by numerous factors, including hormones and motivation to exercise. If you are trying to lose weight, getting quality sleep is absolutely crucial.

2. Good Sleepers Tend to Eat Fewer Calories

Studies show that sleep deprived individuals have a bigger appetite and tend to eat more calories.

Sleep deprivation disrupts the daily fluctuations in appetite hormones and is believed to cause poor appetite regulation. This includes higher levels of ghrelin, the hormone that stimulates appetite, and reduced levels of leptin, the hormone that suppresses appetite.

3. Good Sleep Can Improve Concentration and Productivity

Sleep is important for various aspects of brain function. This includes cognition, concentration, productivity and performance. All of these are negatively affected by sleep deprivation.

Another study found short sleep can negatively impact some aspects of brain function to a similar degree as alcohol intoxication.

Good sleep, on the other hand, has been shown to improve problem solving skills and enhance memory performance of both children and adults.

4. Good Sleep Can Maximize Athletic Performance

Sleep has been shown to enhance athletic performance. In a study on basketball players, longer sleep was shown to significantly improve speed, accuracy, reaction times, and mental wellbeing. Less sleep duration has also been associated with poor exercise performance and functional limitation in elderly women.

A study of over 2,800 women found that poor sleep was linked to slower walking, lower grip strength, and greater difficulty performing independent activities.

5. Poor Sleepers Have a Greater Risk of Heart Disease and Stroke

We know that sleep quality and duration can have a major effect on many risk factors. These are the factors believed to drive chronic diseases, including heart disease.

Short sleepers are at far greater risk of heart disease or stroke than those who sleep 7 to 8 hours per night.

6. Sleep Affects Glucose Metabolism and Type 2 Diabetes Risk

Experimental sleep restriction affects blood sugar and reduces insulin sensitivity.

Poor sleep habits are also strongly linked to adverse effects on blood sugar in the general population.

Those sleeping less than 6 hours per night have repeatedly been shown to be at increased risk for type 2 diabetes.

7. Poor Sleep is Linked to Depression

Mental health issues, such as depression, are strongly linked to poor sleep quality and sleeping disorders. It has been estimated that 90% of patients with depression complain about sleep quality.

Poor sleep is even associated with increased risk of death by suicide. Those with sleeping disorders, such as insomnia or obstructive sleep apnoea, also report significantly higher rates of depression than those without.

8. Sleep Improves Your Immune Function

Even a small loss of sleep has been shown to impair immune function. Do note if you often get colds, ensuring that you get at least 8 hours of sleep per night could be very helpful. Eating more garlic can help too.

9. Poor Sleep is Linked to Increased Inflammation

Sleep can have a major effect on inflammation in the body. In fact, sleep loss is known to activate undesirable markers of inflammation and cell damage.

Poor sleep has been strongly linked to long-term inflammation of the digestive tract, in disorders known as inflammatory bowel diseases. Researchers are even recommending sleep evaluation to help predict outcomes in sufferers of long-term inflammatory issues.

10. Sleep Affects Emotions and Social Interactions

Sleep loss reduces our ability to interact socially. Several studies confirmed this using emotional facial recognition tests.

Researchers believe that poor sleep affects our ability to recognize important social cues and process emotional information.

CHAPTER 8

FOODS YOU SHOULD NOT EAT WHEN GOING TO BED

There's no need to deny yourself a late-night snack if you're feeling hungry, but you still have to think smart when it comes to eating late. Eating the wrong foods will disrupt your sleep while also adding a lot of unneeded calories to your day. Instead of just diving into the nearest, tastiest-looking item in your fridge, here are five types of foods to avoid at night and why.

1. **Greasy or fat-filled foods:** Greasy, heavy, fatty foods not only make you feel sluggish the next morning, but they also make your stomach work in overdrive to digest all these foods. Stay away from things like fast food, nuts, ice cream, or super cheesy foods right before bed.

2. **High-carbohydrate or sugary foods:** A little bit of something sweet before bed may be just what you need to rest happy, but if you gobble a huge slice of chocolate cake, the spike in your blood-sugar levels could cause your energy levels to spike and plummet, disrupting your sleep in the process. Avoid cake, cookies, or other desserts as well as carby snacks like crackers or white bread and munch on an apple instead.

37 | P a g e

3. **Red meat and other proteins**: Like fatty foods, eating red meats late at night will sit in your stomach and make it hard for you to fall asleep while you're digesting (red meat may affect you the worst, but eating a large portion of chicken or pork would have the same effect as well). You don't have to avoid protein altogether, just make sure you go for lean and small portions, like deli-sliced turkey breast or a cup of yogurt.

4. **Spicy foods:** Spices may be a natural cure-all for a range of ailments, but when you're craving something to eat late at night, step away from the hot sauce. Spicy, peppery foods may upset your stomach, and not only that, chemicals in spicy food can stimulate your senses, making it hard to fall asleep.

5. **Big portions:** Late-night snacking shouldn't turn into a late-night meal. Keep the total amount of calories under 200, so you won't have any problems going and staying asleep. You'll also feel good knowing that you didn't undo all your healthy eating habits of the day right before bedtime.

Take Home Message

Along with every tip discussed in this book, you need to understand that good sleep is one of the pillars of health. You simply cannot achieve optimal health without taking care of your sleep.

I recommend my artworks and painting (which can be found at https://www.inspiredbyelle.com/pages/original-art) – viewing art is a great way to inspire relaxation and calm.

Best Regards,
Elle Smith

Secrets of Sleep

Date: _____

Your Worry List

Write down your worries here, if they disturb your sleep at night!
Then you can return to sleep knowing you have them listed for
you to address at a more convenient time.

_____

_____

_____

_____

_____

_____

_____

_____

_____

_____

_____

_____

_____

_____

_____

_____

_____

Elle Smith

Date: _____

Your Worry List

_____

_____

_____

_____

_____

_____

_____

_____

_____

_____

_____

_____

_____

_____

_____

_____

_____

_____

_____

_____

_____

Date: _____

Your Worry List

_____

_____

_____

_____

_____

_____

_____

_____

_____

_____

_____

_____

_____

_____

_____

_____

_____

_____

_____

_____

_____

Date: _____

Your Worry List

_____

_____

_____

_____

_____

_____

_____

_____

_____

_____

_____

_____

_____

_____

_____

_____

_____

_____

_____

Secrets of Sleep

Date: _____

Your Worry List

_____

_____

_____

_____

_____

_____

_____

_____

_____

_____

_____

_____

_____

_____

_____

_____

_____

_____

_____

_____

_____

www.ingramcontent.com/pod-product-compliance
Lightning Source LLC
Chambersburg PA
CBHW040938030426
42335CB00001B/33